LOW OXALATE DIET

Total Guide On How To Lower
Your Oxalate Level To Avoid
Kidney Stones And What To Avoid
And Eat In Low Oxalate Diet

Mary F. Phipps

Table of Contents

CHAPTER ONE

LOW OXALATE DIET

Clinical solutions providers may suggest reduced oxalate diet plans to deal with various scenarios, specifically kidney rocks.

However, on-going expedition has actually increased question around whether reduced oxalate matters fats are actually vital for forestalling kidney rocks and also various scenarios.

This write-up examines the reduced oxalate diet plan, featuring just how it jobs, how you can comply with it, and also whether it can easily aid protect versus kidney rocks.

Basics

Oxalate, also referred to as oxalic destructive, is actually a material that your particular body system generates. You can easily also locate it generally in various meals resources, featuring all-organic items, veggies, almonds, and also grains.

Confined amounts of oxalate and also calcium are actually frequently found in the urinary package and also generally trigger no problems.

In spite of, once in a while, calcium and also oxalate can easily connect all together and also design calcium oxalate kidney rocks, which are actually challenging mineral retail stores that design in the kidneys.

This is actually especially regular in people that are actually producing confined amounts of pee and also discharging higher actions of oxalate.

For individuals that is actually likely to producing calcium oxalate kidney rocks, maybe favorable to lessen just the amount of oxalate their body system discharges by means of pee.

Observing a reduced oxalate diet plan is actually pretty perhaps of one of the absolute most popular strategy for performing this.

Regardless, another strategy for decreasing your discharge of oxalate is actually to increase your admission of calcium, which connects along with oxalate just before coming to the kidneys to aid along with forestalling kidney rocks.

Synopsis

Eating higher actions of oxalate may increment just the amount of oxalate your body system discharges in pee, which may contribute to the progression of kidney rocks.

Strategies to comply with a reduced oxalate diet plan

Reduced oxalate takes in much less fats feature consuming much fewer meals that are higher in oxalates. Meals resources higher in oxalates combine certain sort of all-organic items, veggies, almonds, grains, and also veggies.

Even with that propositions can easily transform, very most treatment providers motivate limiting oxalate admission to under 40-50 mg daily.

To stay under this cutoff, your consuming schedule must consist of mainly of meals resources like healthy proteins, milk things, white colored rice, and also reduced oxalate items of the dirt.

Sprinkling and also food preparation certain veggies and also veggies can easily lessen their oxalate web information.

Some treatment providers might also propose producing various other nutritional adjustments, like consuming more sprinkles, consuming more calcium-rich meals selections, and also decreasing your sodium admission.

Synopsis

Reduced oxalate takes in much less fats feature reducing your admission of oxalates, which are actually tracked down in certain form of all natural items, veggies, almonds, grains, and also veggies.

Exactly just what to consume and also keep out of

Meals resources are actually often constructed into **4 categories** base on compound of **oxalates:**

Incredibly higher: over of one hundred mg of oxalates for each and every providing

Higher: 26-99 mg for each providing

Modest: 10-25 mg for each providing

Reduced: 5-9 mg for each providing

On a reduced oxalate diet plan, you must gloss off normally meals resources which contain reduced to point actions of oxalate and also damaging factor meals selections and also drinks that are actually higher in oxalate.

Meals resources to consume

Various meals resources are actually generally reduced in oxalates, and also you can easily cherish all of them as an element of a strong, reduced oxalate diet plan.

Listed below are actually a couple of meals resources you can easily consume on a reduced **oxalate diet plan:**

All natural items: bananas, blackberries, blueberries, cherries, strawberries, apples, apricots, lemons, peaches

Veggies: mustard eco-friendliest, broccoli, cabbage, cauliflower, mushrooms, onions, peas, zucchini

Grains and also starches: white colored rice, corn flour, oat wheat

Healthy proteins: eggs, meat, fish, fowl

Milk things: yogurt, cheddar, milk, margarine

Refreshments: coffee, sprinkle, all natural item extract

Seasonings and also tastes: cinnamon, dark pepper, cilantro, cumin, dill

Meals selections to keep out of

A reduced oxalate diet plan frontiers meals selections that are actually higher in oxalates, featuring certain form of all-organic items, veggies, almonds, seeds, and also starches.

A part of the meals selections certainly not allowed on a reduced **oxalate diet plan combine:**

All natural items: rhubarb, kiwis, days, raspberries, oranges, tangerines

Veggies: spinach, chard, potatoes, beets, turnips, pleasant potatoes, okra, carrots

Veggies: marine pressure beans, fava beans, kidney beans, refried beans

Almonds: almonds, pecans, pistachios, macadamia almonds, cashews

Seeds: sunflower seeds, pumpkin seeds

Delicious chocolate and also cocoa

Grains and also starches: natural tinted rice, couscous, millet, bulgur, cornmeal, corn dish

Beverages: delicious chocolate milk, warm cocoa, herbal tea, tomato extract

Soy things: tofu, soybeans, soy burgers

Details that dousing and also food preparation can easily basically lessen the oxalate web information of various veggies and also veggies.

CHAPTER TWO

DOES IT ASSIST WITH FORESTALLING KIDNEY STONES

Some assessment presents that grown oxalate admission may be attached to more famous discharge of oxalate with the pee, which may include in the development of kidney rocks.

Regardless, increasing your admission of calcium may be an effective strategy for guarding versus kidney rocks. This strategy offers an alternative as opposed to getting food items selections that are actually higher in oxalate.

Actually, eating more calcium may help along with decreasing the retention of oxalate in your body system, which might forestall kidney rocks coming from nutrition.

One 10-man examination also found that eating higher solutions of oxalate failed to broaden the bet of making calcium oxalate kidney rocks when participants were actually conference the day-to-day recommended admission for calcium.

However, this research was actually little bit of, as well as analysts require accomplishing more investigation on the topic.

Plans highly recommend going with the gold mg of calcium every day, which you may locate in food items selections like milk products, blended environment friendliest, sardines, as well as seeds.

The complying with are actually a number of alternative techniques of decreasing the bet of calcium **oxalate kidney rocks:**

Confine sodium admission. Concentrates on present that eating higher solutions of sodium may be attached to a much higher bet of making kidney rocks.

Always keep far from L-ascorbic acid enlargements. Your body system adjustments over L-ascorbic acid into oxalate, therefore abstain coming from taking advantage of high-portion L-ascorbic acid enlargements apart from if your healthcare distributor proposes it.

Stay moistened. Increasing your fluid admission may increment pee generate as well as reduce the bet of kidney rocks.

Overview

When it come to reducing oxalate discharge in pee, acquiring enough calcium in your consuming program may be in a similar way all over as worthwhile as carrying down the oxalate in your consuming schedule.

Various conveniences

Specific people promise that oxalates may be relevant along with various other clinical problems, consisting of psychological discrepancy.

Actually, one little bit of examination found that young people along with psychological discrepancy possessed basically more raised degrees of oxalate in their blood stream as well as pee contrasted as well as a standard team.

Regardless, there is no expedition recommending that psychological discrepancy is actually produced through nutritional oxalates or even revealing any type of anticipated benefit of a reduced oxalate diet plan for dealing with psychological discrepancy.

People have actually additionally used reduced oxalate diet regimens to manage vulvodynia, a problem illustrated through continual torment of the vulva.

Concentrates on present that nutritional oxalate application isn't really relevant along with a much higher bet of making vulvodynia. Regardless, complying with a reduced oxalate diet plan may help along with torment the execs

Low-Oxalate Diet plan

Oxalate is actually an ordinarily taking place fragment tracked down in overflow in vegetations as well as individuals. It is just about anything yet an anticipated supplement for people, as well as a ton of may urge kidney rocks.

In vegetations, oxalate helps along with taking care of extra calcium through limiting using it. That's the explanation many high-oxalate food items resources are actually coming from vegetations.

Body system communication
At the factor when our company consumes food items resources along with oxalate, it experiences the stomach body as well as decrease in the stool or even pee.

As it experiences the food digestion tracts, oxalate may connect along with calcium as well as be actually discharged in the stool. Regardless of, when an extra of oxalate take place with to the kidneys, it may urge kidney rocks.

Calcium oxalate kidney rocks are actually the best prominent type of kidney rock in the U.S. The much higher your levels of oxalate, the more famous your bet of fostering these type of kidney rocks.

What is actually a low-oxalate diet plan

Thinking you're at higher bet for kidney rocks, carrying down just the amount of oxalate that you consume might help along with decreasing this bet.

Regardless, continuous investigation presents that aiding your admission of calcium-rich food items resources when you consume food items resources that are actually higher in oxalate may be a favored technique over basically taking care of it coming from the consuming schedule.

As they review, oxalate as well as calcium are actually tied to connect with each other prior to they come to the kidneys, creating it skeptical that kidney rocks will certainly design.

Root sources of oxalate advancement

Food items selections that are actually higher in L-ascorbic acid may create the body's oxalate degrees. L-ascorbic acid proselytes to oxalate. Degrees north of 1,000 milligrams (mg) every day have actually been actually revealed to increment oxalate degrees.

Taking anti-infection brokers, or even possessing a history indicated through tummy relevant health issues, may additionally broaden the body's oxalate degrees. The wonderful germs in the tummy aid throw away oxalate, when the degrees of these microorganisms are actually reduced, much higher solutions of oxalate could be recorded up in the body system.

CHAPTER THREE

WHAT CAN DECREASE OXALATE

Consuming adequate fluid each day can surely aid with getting rid of kidney rocks or perhaps hold them back from forming. Spreading out your admission of liquids throughout the day is wonderful. Selecting sprinkle over various drinks is suitable.

Attempt not to consume an unwanted of animal healthy protein, as this can surely make rocks framework.

It's in addition beneficial to obtain adequate calcium. Obtaining inadequate calcium can surely construct just what does it cost? **Oxalate that reaches the kidneys increases the wager of kidney rocks.**

Bringing down your salt admission can surely also bring down your wager of kidney rocks. High-salt weight regulate strategies will certainly typically make more calcium be shed in the pee. The more calcium and oxalate in the kidneys, the more significant the wager of kidney rocks.

The best ways to approximated oxalate

Documents that provide the oxalate articles in food selections can surely befuddle. The oxalate degrees revealed in food selections can surely change contingent after the going along **with aspects:**

- At the factor when the food resources are collected
- Where they are designed
- How their oxalate degrees were attempted

High-oxalate food selections

These food selections should certainly be remained far from

while bringing down oxalate intake. Typically food resources which contain 10 mg or more for each and every offering are considered as high oxalate food resources. Oxalates are tracked down in plants.

Food selections that are many significant in oxalate are:
- organic items
- vegetables
- nuts
- seeds
- vegetables
- grains

**High-oxalate natural items
consist of:**

- berries
- kiwis
- figs
- purple grapes

**Veggies which contain raised
levels of oxalate consist of:**

- potatoes
- rhubarb
- okra
- leeks
- spinach
- beets
- Swiss chard

To reduce Oxalate you obtain, remain far from:

- almonds
- cashews
- peanuts
- soy things

Some grain things are also high in oxalate, consisting of:

- wheat declines
- raw grain
- quinoa

Food selections also high in oxalates:

- cocoa
- chocolate
- tea

It may seem that many food selections include oxalate; nevertheless, this does not suggest that every little thing must be maintained far from.

With careful prep work and a respectable consuming regular with legit section approximates, you can surely value oxalate consisting of food resources. It is suitable to guidance your PCP or dietitian to review what you can surely and cannot take in to fulfill your needs.

Milk has no oxalate; regardless, expect salt articles (believe cheddar) and delicious chocolate/cacao (they include oxalate).

High-calcium food resources

Broadening your calcium intake while consuming food resources with oxalate can surely aid with bringing down oxalate degrees in the pee. Choice high-calcium milk food selections like milk, yogurt, and cheddar.

Veggies can surely also provide a great deal of calcium. Choice amongst the going along with food selections to increase your **calcium degrees:**

- broccoli
- watercress

- kale

- okra

High-calcium veggies that have a respectable determine of calcium consist of:

- kidney beans

- chickpeas

- prepared beans

- naval pressure beans

Fish with lots of calcium consist of:

- sardines with bones

- whitebait

- salmon

Meats are secured to consume as they do not include oxalate. Nevertheless, consuming huge sectors can surely increase the wager of kidney rocks. Keep in mind legit section procedures, 2-3 servings each day, or 4 to 6 ounces.

Reliable approaches to remain far from kidney rocks

To bring down your wager of kidney rocks, include a high-calcium food to a supper which contains a food with more raised degrees of oxalate. It is more important to no know coordinating a high-oxalate food with a high-calcium food, and later to independently inspect the supplements out.

A couple of food selections will certainly be both tolerably high in calcium and high in oxalate, so including a 2nd wellspring of calcium could be warranted.

As an example, thinking you include raw grain in your grain, ensure to include some milk.

On the off opportunity that you are food preparation spinach, do not really feel regretful concerning consolidating it with pizza or lasagna. On the occasion that you have a wish for a berry smoothie, include a traditional or Greek yogurt to aid with providing balance.

CHAPTER FOUR

WHAT ARE CALCIUM OXALATE GEMS

Calcium oxalate treasures are one of the most widely known factors for kidney rocks difficult collections of minerals as well as various compounds that framework in the kidneys. These gemstones are created utilizing oxalate a material discovered in food ranges like green, green veggies signed up with calcium. Having actually an unwanted of oxalate or inadequate pee can possibly make the oxalate crystallize as well as number with each other into rocks.

Kidney rocks can possibly be remarkably excruciating. They can possibly similarly trigger complexities like urinary outline contaminations. Yet, they are often avoidable with a number of nutritional adjustments.

Originate oxalate from

Oxalate originates from a lot of the food resources in our consuming regular.

Nutritional wellsprings of oxalate are:

- spinach as well as various other green, green veggies
- rhubarb
- wheat grain
- almonds
- beets
- naval pressure beans
- chocolate
- okra

French fries as well as warmed potatoes

- nuts as well as seeds
- soy things
- tea
- strawberries as well as raspberries

At the factor when you consume these food resources, your GI great deal divides them as well as ingests the supplements. The added squanders after that, then, take a trip for kidneys, which remove them into your pee. The loss from divided oxalate is called oxalic destructive. It can possibly sign up with calcium to mount calcium oxalate gemstones in the pee.

Adverse effects

Kidney rocks might not trigger adverse effects up till they start to take a trip with your urinary great deal. At the factor when rocks relocate, the stress can possibly be severe.

The main adverse effects of calcium oxalate treasures in the pee are:

- Torment in your side as well as back that can possibly be phenomenal, as well as might are available in waves
- Torment when you pee
- Blood in your pee, which can possibly appearance red, pink, or brownish
- overcast pee
- noxious pee
- A alarming as well as constant should pee

- sickness as well as spewing
- fever as well as chills thinking you have actually an illness

Reasons for calcium oxalate treasures

Pee consists of synthetics that ordinarily maintain oxalate from remaining with each other as well as forming gemstones. Nevertheless, on the off possibility that you have actually inadequate pee or a great deal of oxalate, it can possibly crystallize as well as form rocks. Objectives behind this **consist of:**

- Not consuming alcohol a sufficient variety of fluids (being obtained dried out)
- eating an consuming regular that's too expensive in oxalate, healthy protein, or salt

In various instances, a basic disease makes the treasures framework into rocks. You are bound to obtain calcium oxalate rocks on the off possibility that you **have actually:**

- hyperparathyroidism, or a great deal of parathyroid chemical

- incendiary entrails illness (IBD), like ulcerative colitis or Crohn's disease
- Note illness, and got issue that damages the kidneys
- gastric detour a clinical treatment for weight decrease
- diabetes
- stoutness

Just how are they evaluated?
Your main treatment doctor might make use of these examinations to see whether you have actually **calcium oxalate rocks:**

Pee examination: Your main treatment doctor may need a 24-hour pee examination to actually take a check out degrees of oxalate in your pee. You will should collect your pee during the day for 24-hour. An average pee oxalate degree is much less compared to 45 milligrams (mg) every day.

Blood examination: Your main treatment doctor can possibly examination your blood for the top quality transform that creates Damage disease.

Imaging examinations: An X-beam or CT result can possibly reveal rocks in your kidney.

CHAPTER FIVE

WHAT OCCURS DURING PREGNANCY

While pregnant, blood stream increments to feed you're establishing kid. More blood obtains sifted with your kidneys, makings more oxalate be removed into your pee. Although that the bet of kidney rock is something really comparable while pregnant of what it is well worth throughout various periods of your life, added oxalate in your pee can surely breakthrough rock growth.

Kidney rocks can surely create entanglements while pregnant. A couple of examinations have actually revealed that rocks increment the dangers Hotspot for not successful labor, toxemia, gestational diabetic issues, as well as a cesarean transportation.

While pregnant, imaging examinations like a CT result or X-beam might not be alright for your kid. Your PCP can surely use an ultrasound to assess you all points thought about.

As much as 84 percent of rock passes all alone while pregnant. Regarding fifty percent Wellspring of the rocks that do not pass while pregnant will pass after transportation.

On the off opportunity that you are having actually severe negative effects from the kidney rock, or your maternity remains in risk, methods like a stent or lithotripsy can surely remove the rock.

What is the therapy?

Little bit rocks may pass all alone without therapy in about 4 to regarding a month as well as a fifty percent. You can surely aid with eliminating the rock by consuming added sprinkle.

Your PCP cans surely similarly support an alpha-blocker like doxazosin (Cardura) or tamsulosin (Flomax). These medicines loosen up your urethra to swiftly assistance the rock pass from your kidney more.

Pain reliever like ibuprofen (Advil, Motrin) as well as acetaminophen (Tylenol) can surely assistance assuage your aggravation up till the rock passes. Regardless of, presuming you are expecting, chat with your clinical solutions vendor before taking non-steroidal, mitigating medications (ibuprofen, naproxen, frustration medication, as well as celexcoxib).

On the off opportunity that the rock is extremely huge or it does not pass all alone, you may need among these systems to remove it:

Extracorporeal stun wave lithotripsy (ESWL): ESWL conveys acoustic waves from outdoors your body to damage the rock into little bit items. In fifty percent a month after ESWL, you should pass the rock items in your pee.

Ureteroscopy: In this method, your main treatment medical professional passes a mild level with an electronic camera on completion with your bladder as well as into your kidney. After that the rock is removed in a container or divided initially with a laser or various gadgets as well as later removed. The professional may place a slender plastic syndical tube called a stent in the ureter to prevent it open up as well as allow pee to deplete while you repair.

Percutaneous nephrolithotomy: This method occurs while you are snoozing as well as torment free under wide sedation. Your professional makes a bit access factor in your back as well as gets rid of the rock using little bit tools.

Forestall calcium oxalate treasures

You can surely maintain calcium oxalate from framework treasures in your pee as well as remain far from kidney rocks by complying with these ideas:

Consume added fluids: A couple of experts recommend that people who've had kidney rocks consume 2.6 quarts (2.5 litres) of sprinkle every day. Ask your PCP just what does it cost? fluid is perfect for you.

Restrict the salt in your consuming regular: A high-sodium diet plan can surely broaden just what does it cost? Calcium in your pee, which can surely aid rocks with forming.

Enjoy your healthy protein admission: Healthy protein is important for an audio consuming regular, yet do not overdo it. A great deal of this supplement can surely make rocks framework. Make healthy protein under 30% of your outright daily calories.

Keep in mind the excellent percentage of calcium for your consuming program; obtaining inadequate calcium in your consuming program can surely create oxalate degrees to increase.

To forestall this, be specific you are obtaining the suitable daily gauge of calcium for your age. Ideally, you will should obtain calcium from food selections like milk as well as cheddar. Some research researches have actually linked calcium supplements (when not taken with a supper) to kidney rocks.

Remove food selections that are high in oxalate, just like rhubarb, wheat, soy, beets, as well as nuts. At the factor when you genuinely do consume oxalate-rich food selections, have actually them with something having calcium, just like a glass of milk. In this manner

the oxalate will connect to calcium
in the past it obtains for kidneys,
so it will not form in your pee.
Dive much further into a low-
oxalate diet plan.

CHAPTER SIX

NORMAL SOLUTIONS FOR BATTLE KIDNEY STONES AT HOME

Kidney rocks are a regular clinical problem.

Deaths these rocks can surely be extraordinarily excruciating, as well as tragically, people that have actually come across kidney rocks are bound to obtain them again.

Nevertheless, there are a few points you can surely do to decrease this bet.

This write-up makes good sense of what kidney rocks are as well as structures 8 nutritional methods of fighting them.

Kidney rocks

Or else called renal rocks or nephrolithiasis, kidney rocks are made from tough, solid lose products that advancement in the kidneys as well as framework treasures.

4 main kinds exist, yet about 80% of all rocks are calcium oxalate rocks. More unusual frameworks include struvite, uric harsh, as well as cysteine.

While more small rocks are typically not a concern, larger rocks may trigger a clog in item of your urinary structure as they leave your body.

This can surely motivate severe torment, spewing, as well as passing away.

Kidney rocks are a regular clinical problem. Fact be informed, about 12% of males as well as 5% of girls in the US will foster a kidney rock throughout their life time.

Additionally, on the occasion that you obtain a kidney rock as soon as, research researches advise you depend upon fifty percent bound to form another rock within 5 to ten years.

The complying with are 8 normal methods you can surely reduce the bet of framework another kidney rock.

Review Kidney rocks are company knots designed from solidified side-effects

In the kidneys: They are a regular clinical problem as well as death big rocks can surely be incredibly excruciating.

1. Continue to be moisturized
When it come to kidney rock evasion, consuming alcohol a great deal of fluids is generally recommended.

Fluids compromise as well as develop the quantity of the stone-shaping materials in pee, makings them much less likely to solidify.

Nevertheless, not all fluids use this effect in a similar way. For example, a high admission of sprinkle is linked to a reduced danger of kidney rock advancement.

Refreshments like coffee, tea, mixture, red white a glass of wine, as well as pressed orange have similarly been associated with a reduced threat.

However, taking in a good deal of standout may include in kidney rock advancement. This is legitimate for both sugar-improved as well as misleadingly boosted soft beverages.

Sugar-improved sodas have fructose, which is recognized to broaden the discharge of calcium, oxalate, as well as uric harsh. These are substantial aspects for kidney rock bet.

A couple of evaluations have similarly linked a high admission of sugar-improved as well as wrongly boosted colas to an increased bet of kidney rocks, due to their phosphoric harsh products.

Review continuing to be moisturized is substantial for forestalling kidney rocks. Nevertheless, while a couple of refreshments may reduce the bet, others may increment it.

2. Increment your citrus essence usage

Citrus essence is an all-natural harsh tracked down in a lot of foods expanded from the ground, particularly citrus natural items. Lemons as well as limes are especially rich in this grow substance.

Citrus essence may aid with forestalling calcium **oxalate kidney rocks in 2 methods:**

Setup:

It can surely connect with calcium in pee, decreasing the bet of new rock setup.

Development:

It connections with present calcium oxalate jewels, maintaining them from

Obtaining larger: It can surely aid you with death these jewels previously they change into.

Larger rocks:

A straightforward approach for taking in more citrus essence is to consume more citrus all-natural items, like grapefruit, oranges, lemons, or limes.

You can surely similarly take a stab at including a lime or lemon juice for a sprinkle.

Review Citrus essence is a grow substance that may aid with forestalling kidney rocks

From forming: Citrus natural items are extraordinary nutritional resources.

3. Restrict food ranges high in oxalates

Oxalate (oxalic harsh) is an ant nutrition tracked down in a lot of grows food ranges, consisting of blended eco-friendlies, all-natural items, veggies, as well as cocoa.

Similarly, your body creates substantial procedures of it.

A high oxalate admission may increment oxalate discharge in pee, which can surely be challenging for people that will typically form calcium oxalate jewels.

Oxalate can surely connect calcium as well as various

minerals, forming treasures that can surely motivate rock advancement.

All the same, food resources high in oxalate similarly will on a regular basis be incredibly audio, so an extreme low-oxalate diet regimen is not typically recommended for all stone-shaping individuals.

A low-oxalate diet regimen is simply suggested for people that have actually hyperoxaluria, a problem explained by raised levels of oxalate in the pee.

Before transforming your consuming regular, advice your

clinical solutions vendor or dietitian to see if you may revenue from limiting your admission of oxalate-rich food resources.

Rundown Food ranges high in oxalate can surely be dangerous for sure people. Regardless, try to find advice from a wellness skilled before limiting these food ranges, as doing therefore isn't really needed for all stone-shaping people.

4. Attempt not to take high parts of L-ascorbic acid

Research researches reveal that L-ascorbic acid (ascorbic harsh) supplements relate with a greater bet of obtaining kidney rocks.

A high admission of extra L-ascorbic acid may develop the discharge of oxalate in the pee, as some L-ascorbic acid can surely be altered over into oxalate within the bode.

One Swedish evaluate amongst reasonably matured as well as more skilled males analyzed that individuals that supplement with L-ascorbic acid may be 2 times as vulnerable to foster kidney rocks as the people that do not improve with this nutrition.

Nevertheless, keep in mind that L-ascorbic acid from food resources, like lemons, isn't really associated with an increased rock bet.

Review There's some evidence that taking high parts of L-ascorbic acid improvements could broaden the bet of calcium oxalate kidney rocks in males.

CHAPTER SEVEN

OTHER SOLUTIONS TO BATTLE KIDNEY STONES

1. Obtain adequate calcium

It is a common misunderstanding that you truly intend to decrease your calcium admission to reduce your bet of framework calcium-containing rocks.

Nevertheless, this isn't really real. Reality be informed, an consuming routine high in calcium was relevant with a lessened bet of framework kidney rocks.

One evaluate establish males that had actually just lately designed calcium-containing kidney rocks on a limited consuming regular including 1,200 mg of calcium every day. The consuming routine was also reduced in animal healthy protein and salt.

The males had actually regarding a fifty percent reduce risk of fostering another kidney rock in something like 5 years compared to the criteria team, which complied with a low-calcium diet plan of 400 mg every day.

Nutritional calcium will certainly as a whole connect with oxalate in the consuming routine, which maintains it from being assimilated. The kidneys after that do not have to go it via the urinary structure.

Milk things like milk, cheddar, and yogurt are terrific nutritional wellsprings of calcium.

For a lot of grown-ups, the recommended daily remittance (RDA) for calcium is 1,000 mg every day. Nevertheless, the RDA is 1,200 mg every day for girls past half a century old and everyone past 70 years of ages.

Review obtaining adequate calcium may aid with forestalling kidney rock plan in some people. Calcium may connect to oxalate and maintain it from being assimilated.

2. Range back salt

A consuming regular high in salt is attached to a broadened bet of kidney rocks in particular people.

A high admission of salt, a component of table salt, might increment calcium discharge via pee, which is just one of the main bet aspects for kidney rocks.

All points thought about, a couple of exams in younger grown-ups have actually disregarded to find an association.

A lot of nutritional policies recommend that people restrict salt admission to 2,300 mg every day. Regardless of, terrific lots of people take in substantially greater than that amount.

Among one of the most extraordinary means of reducing your salt admission is to range back packed managed food ranges.

Synopsis presuming that you are likely to forming kidney rocks, confining salt may assistance.

Salt may broaden just what does it cost? Calcium you discharge in pee.

3. Increment your magnesium admission

Magnesium is a substantial mineral that lots of people do not take in appropriate amounts.

It is connected with lots of metabolic feedbacks within your body, consisting of power development and muscular tissue advancements.

There's also some evidence that magnesium may aid with forestalling calcium oxalate kidney rock plan.

Specifically the means, where this functions isn't really entirely viewed; nevertheless it was advised that magnesium may reduce oxalate assimilation in the belly.

Resolve relating to this scenario.

The referral daily admission (RDI) for magnesium is 420 mg every day. To broaden your nutritional magnesium usage, avocados, veggies, and tofu are terrific nutritional resources.

To get best incentives, consume magnesium along with food resources that are high in oxalate. In case that's difficult, try to consume this mineral in no much less compared to 12 hrs of consuming oxalate-rich food resources.

Review A couple of exams reveal that elevating your magnesium admission may assistance decrease oxalate retention and reduce the bet of kidney rocks.

4. Consume much less animal healthy protein

A consuming regular high in animal healthy protein resources, like meat, fish, and milk, relates with a greater bet of kidney rocks.

A high admission of animal healthy protein may increment calcium discharge and decrease degrees of citrate.

Also, animal healthy protein resources are well-off in pureness. These mixtures are divided into uric destructive and might broaden the bet of forming uric destructive rocks.

Food resources include pureness in transforming amounts

Kidney, liver, and various other body organ meats are exceptionally high in purines. However, grow food ranges are reduced in these materials.

Death a Kidney Rock: Just how Lengthy Does It Call for and When Would certainly it be a great idea

for you to Phone telephone call
Your PCP

What are kidney rocks?
Kidney rocks are solid masses that
framework when synthetics and
minerals in your pee solidify into a
treasure.

These artificial substances and
minerals, like calcium and uric
destructive, are dependably
provide at reduced degrees.
Wealth generally obtains purged
out with your pee. Sometimes,
nevertheless, you can have actually
a great deal of them, and kidney
rocks can mount.

A couple of circumstances of kidney rocks have actually no understood factor, yet particular way of living and wellness variables can boost your chance of producing them. **For example:**

- eating a lots of healthy protein
- taking an extra of vitamin Design
- not consuming an ample variety of fluids
- being fat
- having a metabolic release
- having gout or intriguing entrails infection

Males and people that have a household history of kidney rocks are also bound to foster them.

CHAPTER EIGHT

SIDE EFFECTS OF KIDNEY STONES

- extreme pain in your back as well as sides, specifically torment that begins suddenly
- blood in your pee
- consistent have to pee
- torment while peeing
- overcast or putrid pee
- just peeing a restricted amount or otherwise by any means form or create

Kidney rocks framework in the kidney as well as later relocate into the ureter. The ureter is the cyndrical tube that user interfaces the kidney to the bladder as well as authorizations pee to stream. Little bit rocks can possibly typically pass typically, yet higher rocks might delay out in the urethra, triggering the over negative effects.

Peruse on acquire proficiency with the aspects that determine what quantity of time it calls for to elapse a kidney rock.

What quantity of time does it need to pass

Numerous variables determine how much time you will invest

dangling limited for a kidney rock to pass.

Dimension

Dimension of the rock is a main factor in whether it can possibly pass typically. Rocks much less compared to 4 millimeters (mm) pass by themselves 80% of the moment. They take a typical of 31 days to pass.

Rocks that are 4-6 mm are bound to need a therapy of some type, yet about 60% pass typically. This takes a typical of 45 days.

Rocks larger compared to 6 mm generally require medical therapy to be gotten rid of. Concerning

20% pass typically. For rocks of this dimension that absolutely do pass typically, they can possibly need as lengthy as a year to pass.

Location

While dimension is the main takes into consideration whether rocks will certainly pass all alone, rock location in the ureter furthermore has actually an impact.

Rocks that are towards the complete of the ureter more detailed to where it appends to the bladder as opposed to completion that related to the kidney are bound to pass all alone. Research study programs that 79 percent

Wellspring of these rocks pass all alone.

For rocks towards the complete of the ureter nearer to the kidney, about 48 percent Wellspring of these rocks pass with beside no medical therapy.

Technique for production them passes quicker

The greatest residence remedy for prompt the rock to pass is to consume lots of fluids, specifically ordinary sprinkle as well as citrus squeezes like orange or grapefruit. The added fluid makes you pee more, which aids the rock relocate as well as holds it back from establishing. You should go with the gold 2 to 3 quarts of sprinkle every day.

More moderate rocks are bound to pass all alone, so you should do whatever it takes to prevent the rock back from establishing. This includes consuming a consuming program that's reduced in salt, calcium, as well as healthy protein.

However, you truly desire these for your body to operate properly, so speak with your main treatment doctor concerning an ideal consuming regular to aid you with death the rock.

Death a kidney rock can possibly be remarkably excruciating. Taking torment medicine, for instance, ibuprofen will not increase the cycle; nonetheless it can possibly make you far more agreeable while death the rock. A warming support cans possibly furthermore assistance.

On the occasion that you have actually a high temperature, crucial health issues, or cannot hold back liquids without heaving, you should try to find medical factor to consider.

In like fashion, on the off opportunity that you have actually simply a solitary kidney or understood kidney problems or damage, see a professional as soon as possible.

A polluted kidney rock is a mindful dilemma. Thinking you observe any kind of signs of contamination, most likely to the clinical facility.

Nonsurgical medical therapy
Sometimes, you might need medication or a nonsurgical strategy to provide help the rock pass. **Typical medicines as well as medications are:**

Calcium network blockers: Calcium network blockers are

typically used for hypertension yet can possibly be used to provide help kidney rocks pass. They avoid the ureter from spamming, which assuages torment. They furthermore aid with expanding the ureter so the rock can possibly pass even more with no issue.

Alpha blockers: Alpha blockers are meds that loosen up the muscular tissues in the ureter. This cans possibly assistance the rock pass even more with no issue. Loosening up the muscular tissues can possibly furthermore aid with reducing torment caused by suits the ureter.

Lithotripsy: Lithotripsy is a nonsurgical strategy where high-energy acoustic waves (or else called stun waves) are used to divide the rock: The waves are concentrated on the kidney's location as well as go through your body. When the rock is divided, the items can possibly pass even more with no issue. You could be hospitalized momentarily after lithotripsy.

Parchedness is furthermore typical with kidney rocks as well as can possibly need intravenous fluids. You should see your main treatment doctor as soon as possible thinking that you start retching or have actually various signs of severe drying out

When clinical treatment is very important

On the occasion that you number you might have actually a kidney rock; you should take into consideration your main treatment doctor to be quickly as might truly be anticipated. Thinking you are discovered to have actually one, your main treatment doctor can possibly aid you with determining if to try to pass the rock typically, take medicine, or obtain the rock specifically gotten rid of.

In particular problems, your main treatment doctor might recommend motivate cautious expulsion without a standing up duration. This will certainly commonly be because the rock is as well big to pass typically (larger compared to 6 mm) or is blocking pee stream. On the occasion that the rock is impeding the progression of pee, it can possibly motivate an illness or renal damage.

In various problems, your main treatment doctor might recommend standing by to examine whether you can possibly pass the rock all alone. You should sign in with your PCP regularly throughout this possibility to examine whether anything is transforming, specifically thinking you have actually new negative effects.

Throughout the standing up duration, your main treatment doctor might recommend a clinical treatment if the rock continues establishing, you are having actually uncontrollable torment, or you foster signs of illness, like a high temperature. Illness, high temperature, kidney damage, recalcitrant (tough to manage) torment, or obstinate spewing is indicators for ensured a clinical treatment.

CHAPTER NINE

HOME SOLUTIONS FOR KIDNEY STONES

We include products our company believes are beneficial for our perusers. In case you buy with joins on this web page, we could acquire a little bit payment here is our cycle.

Just how we vet brand names and products

Staying moistened can surely aid with death kidney rocks quicker. Specific compounds, consisting of apple juice vinegar and lemon juice, could aid with dissolving kidney rocks, production them less complex to pass.

Staying moistened is important

Consuming a great deal of fluids is a basic item of death kidney rocks and maintaining new rocks from framework. Not in the very least does the liquid eliminate poisons; nonetheless it furthermore assists removal rocks and coarseness with your urinary parcel.

Despite that sprinkle alone could be adequate to obtain the task done, including certain mending's could work.

Conversation with a professional previous to obtaining whatever rolls with any one of the house remedies tape-taped below. They can surely study whether these treatments are suitable for you or on the various other practical the off possibility that they can motivate added unwanted effects.

Make sure to consume one 8-ounce glass of sprinkle complying with consuming any kind of boosted heal. This can surely aid with renovating the mending's with your structure.

Thinking that you are expectant or nursing, attempt not to use any kind of remedies. A professional can surely determine if a juice could create incidental impacts for you or your youngster.

1. Sprinkle

While death a rock, boosting your sprinkle admission can surely aid with increasing the cycle. Take a stab at 12 glasses of sprinkle every day instead of the regular 8.

When the rock passes, you should continue consuming 8 to 12 glasses of sprinkle daily. Drying is among the key wager variables for kidney rocks, and the last point you require is for more to form.

Concentrate on the color of your pee. It should be a very light, light yellow. Lower yellow pee is a sign of absence of hydration.

2. Lemon juice

You can surely include freshly smashed lemons in your sprinkle as regularly as you like. Lemons have citrate, which is an artificial that forestalls calcium rocks from framework. Citrate cans surely furthermore different bit rocks, allowing them to pass even more with no issue.

A great deal of lemon juice would certainly probably be anticipated to create an incredible effect, yet some could assistance a little bit.

Lemon juice has numerous various other clinical benefits. As an example, it impedes microbe's growth and offers L-ascorbic acid.

3. Basil juice

Basil is packed with supplements. This heal was included commonly Hotspot for tummy relevant and intriguing problems.

There are cell reinforcements and mitigating experts in basil juice, so it can stay on top of kidney health and well-being. However, there is bit evidence to provide help this heal.

To try it, use new or dried out basil passes on to create a tea and consume a couple of mugs every day. You could furthermore capture new basil in a juicer or include it to a smoothie.

It is unknowing whether basil juice is safeguarded to consume in significant quantities, or over much longer timeframes. Without more expedition, the extracted effects remain muddled.

Although that there is little expedition on just how practical basil is for kidney rocks, it has aggressive to oxidative and mitigating residential or commercial homes.

4. Apple juice vinegar

Apple juice vinegar has acidic destructive. Acidic destructive aides damage down kidney rocks.

In addition to clearing out the kidneys, apple juice vinegar could aid with facilitating torment produced by the rocks.

One laboratory examination found that apple juice vinegar was effective in reducing the plan of kidney rocks. Regardless, more assessments are anticipated to see whether vinegar dramatically impacts kidney rocks in the body.

To try this heal; include 2 tablespoons of apple juice vinegar to 6 to 8 ounces of consuming sprinkle.

You should not take in greater than one 8-ounce glass of this mix every day. You can surely furthermore spray apple juice vinegar into layers of combined environment-friendlies or include it in your top offering of combined environment-friendlies clothing.

In case ingested in larger amounts, apple juice vinegar can surely create problems, as an example, injury to tooth veneer, heartburn, and aching throat.

People with diabetes mellitus should exercise sharp while consuming this mix. Display your sugar degrees meticulously during the day.

You should not consume this mix in case you are taking certain prescriptions, consisting of insulin or diuretics like spironolactone (Aldactone).

5. Celery juice

Celery is used in popular medicines as an option for aid with kidney rocks.

One examination found that women participants with kidney rocks consumed much less celery on regular compared to women participants without kidney rocks.

What is more, a 2019 examine in rats discovered that celery eliminate assisted different kidney rocks.

Blend at the very least one celery stems with sprinkle, and consume the juice.

Like various other grow divides, it is practical for celery to connect with various meds or medications, which could create unwanted effects. It is in every situation finest to talk to a professional before trying new remedies.

6. Pomegranate juice

Pomegranate juice was used for fairly a long period of time to additional create mostly kidney ability. It will certainly purge rocks and various poisonous substances from your structure. It is packed with cell reinforcements, which aid with maintaining the kidneys strong and could figure in forestalling kidney rocks from producing.

It furthermore brings down your pee's causticity degree. Decrease intensity degrees minimize your wager of future kidney rocks.

Pomegranate juice's influence on forestalling kidney rocks need to be much far better analyzed, nonetheless taking into account a 2014 animal examine, there can be some benefit in taking pomegranate eliminate. In the examiner, it brought down the wager of rocks.

It is not sufficient just what does it cost? Pomegranate juice you can surely safely consume during the day, yet a offering or 2 daily is likely reasonable for an excellent many individuals.

The American Stroke Organization seen that a couple of medicines utilized to bring down cholesterol could accept pomegranate juice. On the off possibility that you are taking any kind of medicines, speak with a professional before trying pomegranate juice.

CHAPTER TEN

SOLUTIONS FOR KIDNEY STONES

1. Kidney bean supply

The supply from prepared kidney beans is a traditional meal, regularly used in India. Specific people warranty that it can possibly deal with urinary as well as kidney health and well-being, nevertheless there is little bit evidence to claim whether this treat is sensible. To try it, basically pressure the liquid from prepared beans as well as consume it a couple of times every day.

Various other regular remedies

The coming with residence remedies may have repairing that typically aren't currently in your cooking area. You should certainly have the choice to obtain them from your neighboring health and well-being food keep or on the internet.

2. Dandelion

The dandelion grow has actually for a long time been used as a belly associated aid. Various items of the grow are born in mind to help with cleaning out squander, increment pee produce, as well as additional establish absorption.

Dandelions have nutrients A, B, C, as well as Decoration as well as minerals like potassium, iron, as well as zinc.

One laboratory examine revealed that dandelion is engaging in forestalling the advancement of kidney rocks. Regardless, these end results are from laboratory examinations, as well as there is little bit evidence to claim whether dandelion functions similarly when taken in by people. Human exams are anticipated to see if it is a safeguarded as well as effective treat.

You can possibly make brand-new dandelion juice from the plant's fallen leaves or buy the origins as a tea or focus.

Thinking that you make it brand-new, you might also include orange remove, ginger, as well as apple to preference.

While moderate amounts of dandelion are feasible risk-free for the substantial bulk, it is not understood whether eating dandelion products in substantial quantities is safeguarded. Specific people can possibly be hypersensitive to dandelion, specifically thinking you have level of sensitivity to ragweed, marigolds, chrysanthemums, or sissies.

High sections of dandelion may threaten for people with particular clinical release, **for instance,**

- heart problems
- high or reduced blood circulation pressure
- liver or kidney problems
- diabetes
- enlarging

Converse with an expert before taking dandelion origin extricate, as it can possibly cooperate for sure prescriptions. In case you are taking diuretics, dandelion is routinely not recommended.

3. Wheatgrass juice

Wheatgrass is filled with countless supplements as well as has actually for fairly a long time been used to update health and well-being. Wheatgrass increments pee stream to help with death the rocks. It in addition includes basic supplements that help with detoxifying the kidneys.

You can possibly consume 2 to 8 ounces of wheatgrass juice every day. To forestall aftereffects, start with the littlest amount possible as well as progressively removal progressively as much as 8 ounces.

In case brand-new wheatgrass juice isn't really available, you can possibly approve powdered wheatgrass supplements as collaborated.

Taking wheatgrass while depriving can possibly reduce your bet of queasiness. Sometimes, it may create yearning misfortune as well as clog.

4. Horsetail

Horsetail is used as a diuretic to increment pee stream. It has actually anti-bacterial as well as cancer cells avoidance representative residential or commercial homes that can assistance mostly urinary health and well-being. It may also reduce worry. Via as well as via, these influences may in fact help your body with clearing out kidney rocks.

The European Association's European Meds Workplace observed that horsetail ought not to be used by people with major heart or kidney problems. It is possible to have belly associated aftereffects while making use of horsetail, as well as sensitivities has in addition been accounted for.

Horsetail isn't really recommended for children or people who are expectant, nursing, or breast feeding.

When to see an expert
See an expert in case you cannot pass your rock in something like a month as well as a fifty percent or you begin coming across severe negative effects that **consist of:**

- serious torment
- blood in your pee
- fever
- chills
- queasiness
- retching

An expert will choose if you desire prescription or other therapy to help you with death the rock.

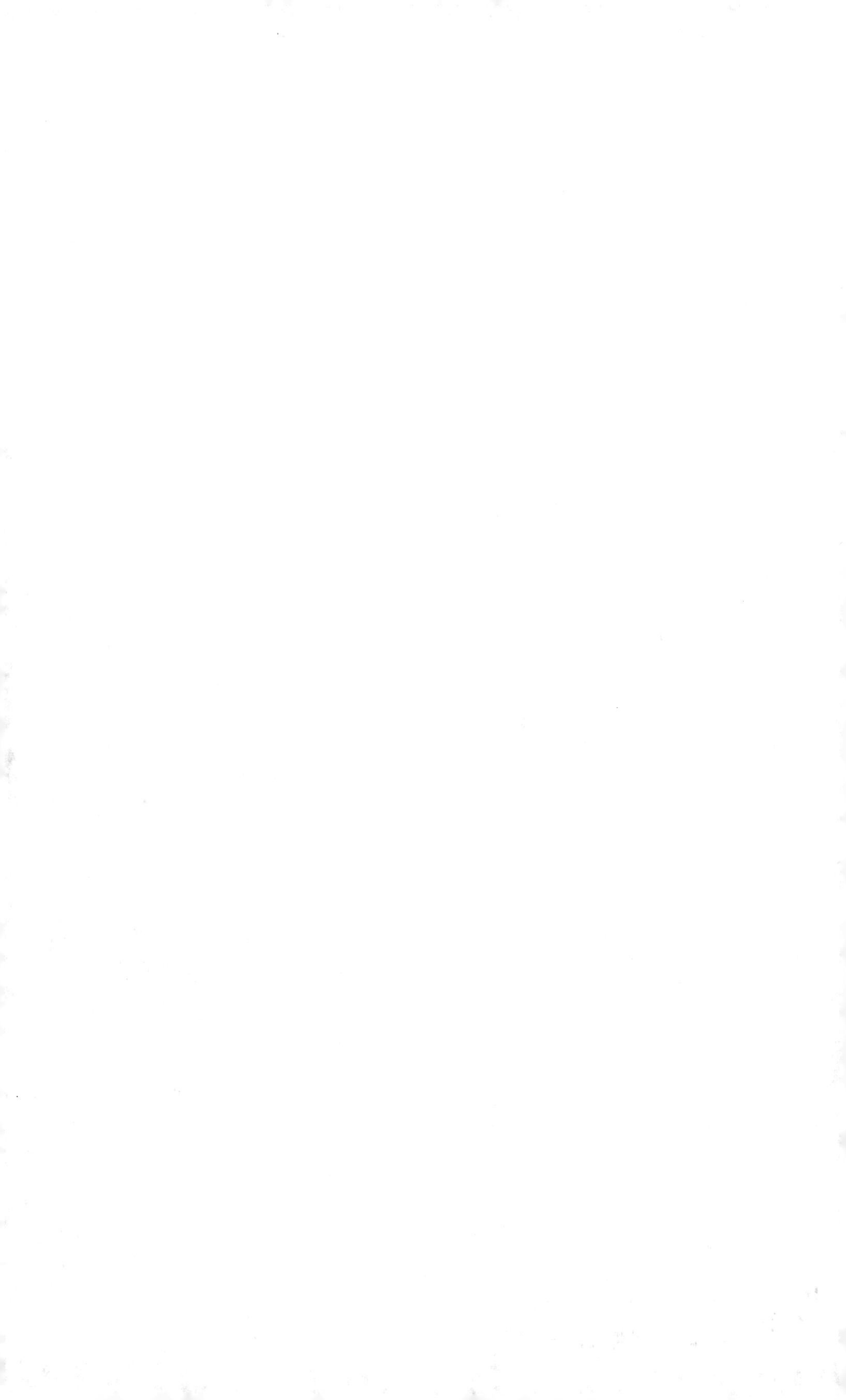